FAQs about How To Eat To Live

Frequently Asked Questions

Volume I

Kevin A. Muhammad

TechDoc, Incorporated
Newark, Delaware

FAQs About How To Eat To Live, Volume I
by Kevin A. Muhammad

Published in the United States by:
TechDoc, Incorporated
7 Waltham Street
Newark, Delaware 19713
Web site address: http://www.etechpublish.com/

Book design by Kevin A. Muhammad
Cover design by Kevin A. Muhammad, Jr.

Printed in the United States of America.
Main entry under title:
FAQs About How To Eat To Live: Volume I

A TechDoc book
graphics; p. 72

Library of Congress Card No. 2002093823
ISBN: 0-9658864-5-X

Meaning of Book Cover

All volumes in this series, *FAQ's About How To Eat To Live*, have the same foundational cover design—with the cover of *How To Eat To Live* placed as a watermark on the front cover, and the image of *clocks* placed on the back cover. Both images represent the essence of this series.

As the ultimate goal of this series is to support and promote the dietary guidance provided by the Honorable Elijah Muhammad in the books *How To Eat To Live (books 1 & 2)*, it is befitting to include this watermark image on the cover of every volume. And, because the essential principle of this divine dietary guidance is to regulate our food intake at 24-hour cycles, the *clock* image is best suited to represent this principle.

Appreciation

All Praise and Honor Belongs to Almighty Allah (God), Who Came in the Person of Master Fard Muhammad, the Great Mahdi, for Giving Humanity Divine Guides in the Persons of the Honorable Elijah Muhammad and the Honorable Minister Louis Farrakhan.

Special thanks to my beloved family: wife, Marcia; and children, Kevin, Jr., and Krystina for their great love and support.

Dedication

To the members of the human family who seek to know and learn of the correct diet for humans; and who are in pursuit of optimum health and longevity. This book is a testimony of the Guidance that can help achieve those outcomes, *How To Eat To Live, (books 1 & 2)*, written by the Honorable Elijah Muhammad. I advise everyone to read and follow this Divine Dietary Guidance.

These books by Kevin A. Muhammad
are available at various outlets.
Visit **www.etechpublish.com** for more information.

Obesity, Diabetes and How To Eat To Live

Nuts Are Not Good for Humans: Biological Consequences of Consumption

The Slave Diet, Disease & Reparations

Whose Protein? The Value of the Soybean and Navy Bean to Human Nutrition: A Comparative Study

Preface

In the Name of Allah, The Beneficent, The Merciful
I Bear Witness There Is No God But Allah,
I Bear Witness Muhammad is His Messenger

Two things inspired the idea of a book comprised of questions and answers about *How To Eat To Live*, the divine dietary guidance of the Honorable Elijah Muhammad. First, my desire to understand this guidance, specifically why we have been instructed to eat as described, has led me to research many points presented by the Honorable Elijah Muhammad. Such activity has been and continues to be very edifying. In presenting this research, I have written articles and books, and have given lectures about the value of this dietary guidance. Some of this research is presented in this book.

The second motivation is to propagate this divine dietary guidance, as the solution to the long-standing health crises faced by this nation and the world. This, of course, is a tremendous goal, and certainly requires great efforts by scores of like-minded people. Although my personal effort toward this goal is edifying, I know that by joining with others who are endeared to this same goal, we can make recognizable progress.

My belief has been that further research into the divine dietary instructions offered by the Honorable Elijah Muhammad can serve as a platform for unity and progress towards the goal of improving the overall health of the world's population. This effort would also increase appreciation for this life-giving and life-saving guidance, halting the inconsistent adherence to this dietary practice that have caused some to confront diseases and illnesses that this dietary guidance is meant to prevent. Greater research can foster a more matured understanding, which can benefit those who know, as well as those who yet do not know.

Finally, in the Holy Quran, Allah states:

And if all the trees on earth were pens and the ocean (were ink), with seven oceans behind it to add to its (supply), yet would not the words of Allah be exhausted (in the writing): for Allah is Exalted in Power, full of Wisdom. (Holy Quran 31:27)

This passage represents my sentiments with respect to this book. Therefore, this book, *FAQs About How To Eat To Live, Volume 1,* represents a humble effort to briefly explain the reasons we have been told to eat as described in *How To Eat To Live.* These explanations are in no way exhaustive, as books can be written to answer each question contained in this volume.

I pray Allah that these explanations will be of some value to the reader.

Table of Contents

Introduction

The books *How To Eat To Live (books 1 & 2)* presents us with many extraordinary aspects, two of which are pertinent to this book. First, the dietary guidance provided by the Honorable Elijah Muhammad is astoundingly logical and simple. The fundamental principles that ensure health and longevity are provided in a most simplistic way that even an absolute fool cannot honestly declare that he or she does not understand. Additionally, this guidance is contained in two books or volumes, which combined, are slightly over 300 pages.

As elementary as these "props" may seem, they are of the utmost importance. Mass confusion does not only persist in the health arena on a wide scale, but many health and nutrition books are filled with obscurities, inconsistencies and contradictions. Many of these books are in upwards of 500 or 600 pages, leaving the reader fatigued and confused. Therefore, to have the principles that support health very clearly explained, using few words, is something that most people eagerly welcome.

Of course, the simplicity of the dietary guidance offered in *How To Eat To Live* should not suggest that our effort to follow this guidance is easy. One's will power is significantly challenged because this dietary guidance is directly opposed to mainstream dietary thought and practices. For example, we are exhorted to move from eating four to five meals a day (or from eating all day long), which are the norms in this society, to eating only once a day. Such a dramatic change affects every aspect of a person's life.

The things we eat and the manner in which we eat them are intrinsic to our social and cultural behaviors; therefore, any knowledge that radically changes our dietary habits directly changes our social and cultural behavior, especially a diet that is profoundly integrated into our belief in Almighty God. Therefore, anyone making an effort to follow the guidance in *How To Eat To Live* should expect varying levels of difficulty, including setbacks. However, persistency will make this dietary guidance easier to practice. The person will become increasingly comfortable with this new diet.

Secondly, the claims made by the Honorable Elijah Muhammad—the expected results of following His guidance are very extraordinary. For example, in one statement, He claims that He can make a child live 240 years by feeding it a diet consisting of navy bean soup. In another statement, He claims that we can live a disease-free life, never getting sick or ill. Whether we believe Him or do not believe Him, these claims should inspire some investigation.

We must keep in mind that when it comes to dietary guidance, the best investigation comes from one's practice of that guidance. To dismiss His claims without ever attempting to prove them right or wrong is unintelligent and disqualifies that person's judgment. Too many people have this ignorant mindset.

The improvement in one's health through the practice of this dietary guidance gives us a glimpse into the truth of the greater claims. It shows that we are on the road to achieving the greater claims. However, because the greater claim—living disease-free for 120, 140, 240 or more years—rests in our consistency in practicing this diet, we must remain focused and enthusiastic. Our approach must become more scientific and less emotional. This compels us to dig deeper into the truths and discover why we are benefiting as we are from this guidance.

For those who have reached this point, further research into this guidance will allow us to truly learn about ourselves in every respect, and give us a greater appreciation for the sciences and laws that govern life. Is this philosophical mumbo-jumbo? No. The true premise for scientific discovery is based on man's quest to live the life preordained by God, which includes living long and disease-free.

Life sciences, such as biology, chemistry, and biochemistry, to name a few, are employed to improve the quality and longevity of human life, and not to destroy human life. Unfortunately, this is not the case with mainstream scientists and scientific institutions. Because of their quests for profit, science is used to concoct pills and potions, and not to support the natural orders or processes setup by God. One such process is the requirement that humans eat food to maintain life.

Science should be used to demonstrate how a specific dietary regimen could achieve results that are out of the reach of any pill or potion. These results are the achievement of far longer lifespans than what is currently being achieved. The sad thing is that too many people believe in miracle pills and potions as a means to achieve optimum health. In his book, *Megatrends*, John Naisbitt, writes:

> We are always awaiting the new magical pill that will enable us to eat all the fattening food we want, and not gain weight; burn all the gasoline we want, and not pollute the air; live as immoderately as we choose, and not contract either cancer or heart disease.
>
> In our minds, at least, technology is always on the verge of liberating us from personal discipline and responsibility. Only it never does and it never will. The more high technology around us, the more the need for human touch.

Very beautifully put! The extremely challenging situations humans have faced through the annals of time demonstrate our awesome power to adapt. This power is innate. All of us have been required to function under difficult situations. Some people have no arms. Some have no feet. Some are mentally disabled. However, in all cases, humans demonstrate a remarkable ability to adapt to difficult circumstances through personal discipline and responsibility. So, in truth, we can never evade our birthright. Unfortunately, our attempt to do so has caused us great harm, and has now endangered our very existence.

Despite this fact, mainstream medical scientists and commercial industries continue their erroneous quests. Moreover, although we complain, we are continuing our quest to promote disease-free living and longevity by encouraging personal discipline and responsibility through the practice of divine dietary guidance. The foremost step in this effort is to become thoroughly acquainted with this divine dietary guidance. This book, *FAQs About How To Eat To Live*, is a part of this quest.

Some might ask, "Why a book of questions and answers about *How To Eat To Live*"? Actually, the raising of questions is in keeping with the mandate given by the Honorable Elijah Muhammad. He has constantly encouraged us to question Him, and not to accept His Teachings on face value. This challenge was not pompously rendered, as if to imply that He gets joy out of proving us wrong. Not so! This was and is for our benefit. It is difficult to appreciate or value something without looking deeper into it. The more we seek to validate knowledge by digging deeper into it, the more we appreciate its value for improving our lives. Questioning is the process that enables us to mine the depths of knowledge.

Additionally, the Honorable Elijah Muhammad wants to mature us. A bad characteristic of ignorant people is that they are prone to accept the words of others, whom they perceive as superior, on face value. Black people (especially the ex-slaves of America) epitomize this syndrome of ignorance. Traditionally, we have never questioned the knowledge, training, instructions, or guidance of our slavemasters, as well as those who currently rule. We accepted their guidance on face value, only to find ourselves plummeting further into the darkness of ignorance, not having the power to do anything beneficial for ourselves.

So, having been presented with a totally new way of life, in every facet, through the Teachings of the Honorable Elijah Muhammad, some people, due to ignorance, have opted to reject these Teachings because they are contrary to most, if not all, traditional and contemporary customs and norms. Some people have done this without examining the results of that which they have ignorantly accepted and practiced.

Such examination would seem most appropriate in light of the fact that mayhem and disease afflicts nearly every household in America. However, the thing that has made self-examination difficult is our adoption of norms and traditions that go hand-and-hand with disease, mayhem, and death. The Teachings of the Honorable Elijah Muhammad challenges these traditions and norms by presenting a nearly "unbelievable" set of values—in every respect—to replace them. The bar is raised beyond our imagination.

If we are courageous enough to examine the Teachings of the Honorable Elijah Muhammad through scientific questioning and research, then we can better examine those set of norms and traditions that we have followed, and confront the reality, which is the uselessness of these traditions in giving us life and life more abundantly.

Again, before being enlightened through the Teachings of the Honorable Elijah Muhammad, Black people never truly questioned the quality and validity of the training we received from our former slavemasters and their children. We never blamed our poor health status on the slave diet that was forced upon us. Now, we are looking carefully into this training, and are uncovering many shocking realities. One such reality is that we are no healthier, as a people, today, than we were while enslaved on the plantation.

In the dietary guidance given by the Honorable Elijah Muhammad, we have been given something that boast good health and longevity. This is clearly stated in *How To Eat To Live*. However, with respect to our former slavemasters and their children, at what point did they claim that the slave diet would give us good health and longer life? They never made such a claim and will never make that claim. So, what right do we really have to reject the Honorable Elijah Muhammad's guidance?

Again, the nature of claims made by the Honorable Elijah Muhammad in *How To Eat To Live* should stimulate some level of curiosity. For many, they have done just that, and this curiosity has given rise to many questions. Through questions, we are able to obtain answers that improve our lives. And, questions that pertain to health, diet and nutrition—which work to sustain our lives—are among the most valuable questions to ask. Through questioning the dietary guidance and laws presented in *How To Eat To Live*, we will discover rich insights into the sciences and laws that govern our lives.

This volume of *FAQs About How To Eat To Live* is the first of many to come, Allah Willing. In this volume, we have selected questions designed to plumb deeper into the framework of this dietary guidance. This volume poses questions about the Source of this Guidance (Question 1), and about the Instructions that represent the pillars of health and longevity (Questions 2 through 9). The answers given are very brief and serve the purpose of stimulating thought and discussion.

1

From God In Person, Master Fard Muhammad

Why does the cover of How To Eat To Live read: "From God In Person Master Fard Muhammad"?

The obvious answer is that *Master Fard Muhammad is the source of the content contained in these books.* The Honorable Elijah Muhammad has emphatically established this throughout both books (*How To Eat To Live, books 1 & 2*), as he wants us to know where, precisely, this dietary guidance has its origin. Given the importance of food in sustaining health, we should want to know who authorizes the dietary recommendations or guidance that we follow.

The term *authorize* does not merely refer to the freedom that any person has to offer dietary guidance, as millions of people have done and continue to do. Authorize, in this context, is the source of the knowledge that supports this dietary advice. In a more direct sense, through whose authority does anyone render dietary advice? What makes that person qualified to give dietary advice? By what means does one judge or measure these qualifications?

If we search this nation's libraries and bookstores, we will find thousands, if not millions, of diet-related books. It seems that everyone wants to add his or her two-cents to this subject, which we must admit, has created mass confusion and caused millions of people to suffer. Surveys have shown that the public is growing more confused and frustrated about dietary advice.[1] Contradictions and falsities have convoluted the nutrition field. Some people are opting to not bother with the issue at all. They would rather eat the foods they like and suffer the consequences. This resolve is among the reasons for the chronic disease epidemic. Although this frustration is understandable, people should continue to seek the true knowledge of nutrition and diet.

---

1. Ruth E. Patterson, P., RD, et al., Is there a consumer backlash against the diet and health message? Journal of the American Dietetic Association, 2001. 101(1): p. 37.

In this debacle of mass confusion and competition, many people yearn for the true advice or guidance—which is supreme among all. Who can give the best and perfect advice about diet other than Almighty God, Himself? Moreover, because all of us eat, we should want to know whether the guidance we are following is from Almighty God or someone else. In the truest sense of this consideration, we can only follow two paths of guidance—Almighty God's or *fallen* man's. These are the only two sources of guidance for human beings.

The risk associated with following *fallen* man is that people will find themselves victimized by ploys that support someone's low and selfish desires to make money. These ploys include, but are not limited to, issuing false advice and marketing poisonous products, including poisonous foods. Almighty God is interested in providing us with the best. He is also interested in uncovering falsehood so that people will have the chance to avoid the pitfalls that destroy their lives.

There are some diets offered by people who claim that such diets are from God, and represent the diets of those who lived during Biblical times. To their credit, at least, these persons have considered God in their diets; however, they have done so in a very limited way.

Part of this limitation is their lack of knowledge about the dietary practices of those who lived 5,000 or more years ago. For example, the Scriptures of both Bible and Holy Quran clearly demonstrate that God is interested in man's diet, as indicated in the dietary laws mandated for the Children of Israel. However, the Scriptures do not provide information about the precise foods eaten by those who had lifespans of 400, 500 or 900 years, such as Noah and Methuselah, or about how they prepared the foods they ate.

Additionally, the Scriptures provide no information about the frequency in which these great patriarchs ate their meals. Anyone who is serious about offering the "Biblical diet" must have these details or they are merely conjecturing, which is no different from what many so-called health experts now do. For the most part, mainstream and new age diets are based on assumptions and conjectures. There is little, if any, power in assumptions or conjectures to produce positive results. The chronic disease epidemic is proof enough to support this statement.

Another part of this limitation is their belief that God is not real or human, which billions of people, including many theologians also believe. This makes their attempt to offer the "Biblical diet" fall extremely short. Only Almighty God can share with us the precise diet of those who lived hundreds of years. According to the Scriptures, He does this when He comes to setup His Eternal Kingdom—in the Last Days. This fact is firmly established in the Holy Quran and Bible. The Gospel of John records that when the Messiah comes, He will give the people *life and more life abundantly.* The Honorable Elijah Muhammad states that the Bible does not describe how he would do this, but declares that such could not be possible unless that One taught us how to eat in such a way that the result would extend our lives, enabling us to avoid disease and premature death.

The Scriptures also provide the reasons why man's lifespan was reduced to its current span of 70 or so years. In Genesis, Almighty God states that because of man's persistent evil imagination, He reduced the human lifespan to 120 years.[2] This was a curse. No longer would man live the length of 500, 800, or 900 years. Later, in Psalm 90, the Prophet David writes:

The length of our days is seventy years or eighty, if we have the strength; yet their span is but trouble and sorrow, for they quickly pass, and we fly away.

Is this not what most people confront today? Is not the average lifespan a mere 70 or 80 years? Does not emotional and physical troubles and sorrow fill these 70 or 80 years?

Knowing that the evidence that proves Almighty God's arrival in the Last Days would be the increased lifespan and improved quality of life of those who follow His guidance, those who are serious about recognizing the signs of His arrival must look for someone issuing a dietary law that has as its ultimate aim, the substantial increase of human lifespan. This is the precise teaching offered in *How To Eat To Live.*

Some people have balked at the words *God In Person, Master Fard Muhammad.* These people are offended because the word "God" refers to a specific person, who has a specific name. For some, their emotions have led them to view *How To Eat To Live* in an improper light. Those who feel

---

2.   Genesis 6:3-6. In: C.I. Scofield DD, ed. The Holy Bible. New Scofield Reference Edition ed. New York: Oxford University Press, 1967.

this way have done themselves a grave disservice. Despite the Scriptural passages that show that God is a human being, many continue to hold on to the falsehood that He is a spirit. Where do they get such notions, when the Scriptures say otherwise?

Those who believe that Almighty God is a human being and that every eye shall see Him, must turn their attention to certain realities, some of which are evident in their lives. For example, should not Almighty God have a name to Himself? Are we to just call him *God* when we see Him? Is *God* His personal name? If it is, then why is not our name *god* too, since we are all *gods*, children of the Most High God?

The word god means power and force, and Almighty God is that human being who exerts unmatched, unequalled and supreme power and force. As lesser gods, we also exert power and force. The Almighty God, however, can easily overcome our power.

Now consider this. As little gods, we have personal names, such as James, David, and Ruth. Why should not the Most High God have a personal name, such as Fard? Furthermore, if we are all beings, having personal names, then why should not the Supreme Being (which makes Him the Almighty God) have a personal name, too? In the book, *Message to the Blackman In America*, the Honorable Elijah Muhammad tells us why Almighty God chose the name Fard for Himself.[3] This name has great meaning and is evidence of the Messiah's arrival. The Honorable Elijah Muhammad also provides Biblical and Quranic passages that prove that Almighty God is a human being.

In completing the answer to this question, two passages from the Bible and Holy Quran, respectively, are presented. These verses, undoubtedly, show that God's interest in man's diet is because He, too, is a human being and therefore, must eat, as do other human beings. This not only confirms His interest in diet, but also establishes the fact that He prescribes our diet.

These verses describe the Prophet Abraham's interaction with God. In Genesis 18: 1-10, we read:

(1) Then the LORD appeared to him by the terebinth trees of Mamre, as he was sitting in the tent door in the heat of the day. (2) So he lifted his eyes and looked, and behold, three men were

---

3.   Muhammad E. Message To The Blackman In America. Chicago: FCN Publishing Co., 1965.

standing by him; and when he saw them, he ran from the tent door to meet them, and bowed himself to the ground, (3) and said, "My Lord, if I have now found favor in Your sight, do not pass on by Your servant. (4) Please let a little water be brought, and wash your feet, and rest yourselves under the tree. (5) And I will bring a morsel of bread, that you may refresh your hearts. After that you may pass by, inasmuch as you have come to your servant." They said, "Do as you have said."

The context of this passage was that God, accompanied by two of His angels, came to inform Abraham that He had decided to destroy Sodom and Gomorrah, and that Lot and his family and followers would be the only people spared.

How would any of us treat Almighty God, if He came to visit with us? Would we not offer Him food and drink? Of course, we would. We might also be nervous about offering Him the right food, knowing (or, at least assuming) that He would not eat just anything. There might be things in our cupboards that we know He would not eat. Abraham played it safe by offering Him bread. The point is that God eats, and therefore, must possess the best dietary knowledge of all. We just cannot imagine Almighty God eating filth, such as pig feet, or drinking whiskey.

The Holy Quran 37:89-93 records a wonderful account of Abraham's knowledge of God's reality. [4] It reads:

[Abraham said] (87) What is then your idea about the Lord of the worlds? (88) Then he glanced a glance at the stars, (89) And said: Surely I am sick (of your deities). (90) So they turned their backs on him going away. (91) Then he turned to their god and said: Do you not eat? (92) What is the matter with you that you speak not? (93) So he turned upon them, smiting with the right hand.

This puts this subject in greater perspective, while demonstrating that the Holy Quran, indeed, verifies the truths contained in the Bible. Abraham knew a God, who ate and spoke, and not a god made by man's hands or a mystery god that cannot be seen, the latter two of which can do nothing to serve humanity.

Finally, the Scriptures teach us that Almighty God has sent various instructions to guide humans back to the right path. In many cases, their

---

4.   Chapter 37 'Al-Saffat' (Those Ranging In Ranks). The Holy Quran. 7 ed. Ohio: Ahmadiyyah Anjuman Ishaat Islam, 1991;859

entire way of life was wrong—diet, proper human relationships, economics, etc.

The Honorable Elijah Muhammad has constantly declared that the Coming of this One, Master Fard Muhammad, is the fulfillment of the Scriptures—both Holy Quran and Bible. These books prophesy of the coming of God in the Last Days to save His people, destroy the wicked, and setup an eternal kingdom.

In doing this, the Scriptures state that He Will give us the Truth that will make us free. He will inform us of many things that we did not know. In short, He will reveal all truth. It is rather obvious that man and mankind do not have this *all truth* because the dangerous time in which we live is the result of that which has governed this world—an over abundance of falsehood, and very little truth, if any at all.

Reasonably, this *all truth* must encompass every human endeavor—health, science, medicine, economics, and politics. The Bible teaches that a government will be upon the Son of Man's shoulders. A government is an institution that serves as the platform for handling the needs of the people. What are our needs? Well, the most common needs are food, shelter, and clothing; and because millions of people are hungry, naked, and out of doors, it is reasonable to assume that He will have to correct these conditions. And, if He is to provide food, then He certainly must provide dietary guidance to ensure that we live long and healthy lives. This guidance is contained in the books, *How To Eat To Live (books 1 & 2)*.

2

Eating the Proper Foods

The Honorable Elijah Muhammad constantly exhorts us to eat the proper foods. What are the proper foods?

This question might seem a bit trite, but how many of us have thought very carefully about the things or qualities that make one food proper and another food improper? If answered honestly, many would have to admit that the word "proper" hardly comes to mind when we eat food or the things we call food. This is not our fault. We are not trained to think meticulously about subjects that address the proper maintenance of our lives.

The educational institutions that provide dietary guidance do so without meticulous consideration or knowledge about the foods they recommend. They offer assumptions and guidance based on conjectures; and when things go wrong, such as the health crisis currently wrecking havoc on us, they bombard us with epidemiological studies that tell us just how bad we are doing. Even in this, they never accept responsibility for this mess. This is the reason why poor health continues as a national epidemic.

In *How To Eat To Live,* the Honorable Elijah Muhammad points out those foods that are proper for us to eat, as well as the foods that are unfit for human consumption. Anyone who has examined the latter knows that it contains most, if not all, of the foods we have been accustomed to eating.

Therefore, the answer to this question will not contain this information. In answering this question, we will focus on the purpose for food. Many people will opt to select foods not mentioned in *How To Eat To Live.* Therefore, some knowledge about how best to view food will enable us to select foods that are fit for human consumption.

What is the purpose of food? As a backdrop for this answer, let us consider the following. The earth is a living entity, and because all life comes from the earth, life depends upon the earth, in many respects, for support. As living organisms, we are in a constant state of motion. This motion brings about a constant need for restoration, revitalization, replenishing, and regeneration. The new replacing the old is life's most constant process. Food provides the cell with the material needed to revive, replenish, regenerate, and restore it. And, because our bodies are made from the earth, we eat material from the earth to sustain ourselves. Let us go further.

We know from our biology lessons that the body cells, although arranged in tissues, are the basic units that make up the body. The cell's most essential processes are self-maintenance and reproduction. Cells are maintained by regenerating any components that become damaged or are turned over by normal cellular processes. Cell reproduction requires energy to complete its reproduction processes. To carry out these chores on a continuous basis the cell requires energy—in the form of substances that serve as fuel. These substances or nutrients also supply the cell with structural materials needed to replenish it. This is precisely what food is designed to accomplish.

Food is generally defined as *material consisting essentially of water, protein, carbohydrate, fat, vitamins and minerals used in the body of an organism to sustain growth, repair, and vital processes and to furnish energy.* Much more can be stated about this definition. For example, based on the state of the body, food can be required for growth (as with children), repair (due to disease or illness), or to furnish energy for sustenance (in the case of both children and adults). Our diets should be driven by these conditions.

This food gets to us through the process of digestion. The digestive process takes the ingested food and degrades it to the state wherein the cells can properly use it. The success of this process depends on the type of food consumed, as well as the overall condition and functionality of the digestive organs.

So, food is a necessity of life for every creature on the earth. All creatures depend upon food to maintain themselves. However, each creature has food designed specifically for it. It is in this area where grave mistakes are made, as assumptions take precedence over facts; and the quest for money via bogus dietary advice takes precedence over sincere and exhaustive efforts to determine the proper foods.

With respect to proper foods for humans, the prevailing assumption is that humans can eat just about anything—from bugs to wood. Within this range of so-called food are many indigestible and harmful materials. Therefore, if the true reason for eating is to sustain our lives by providing the body with the proper nutrients, eating harmful foods does not achieve this.

According to The Random House College Dictionary, the term "proper" is defined: *1)...adapted or appropriate to the purpose or circumstances; fit; suitable 2) conforming to established standards or behavior or manners; correct or decorous 3) belonging to or pertaining to a particular person or thing.* Proper foods are foods that provide humans with essential nutrients. Proper foods are foods easily degraded and assimilated by the digestive tract. There is yet more to this, as the Honorable Elijah Muhammad has pointed out that proper foods cannot only be determined by their nutritional content but also by the amount of poisons contained in them when they are in both their raw and processed (cooked) stages.

A prevailing and most destructive dietary assumption is that raw foods— vegetables and meat—are best for health. With respect to vegetables, many nutritionists believe that cooking vegetables will reduce their nutritional value, as cooking will remove some vitamins, minerals and other nutrients. This is emphatically incorrect. Cooking improves the nutritional value of vegetables, as this value is not measured quantitatively but qualitatively. I would rather eat a cooked vegetable that contains 75% digestible nutrients and no poison, than eat a raw vegetable that contains 100% indigestible and poisonous nutrients.

Most vegetables contain complex nutrients that are very dense, meaning they are comprised of various types of chemical bonds. These bonds must be broken or made permeable through the action of heat. In this state, the digestive enzymes are most effective at completing the process of degrading the food to its basic units. Therefore, cooking (i.e. boiling, autoclaving, etc.) is an essential step in preparing vegetables for human consumption.

Eating raw meat should be out of the question. Some people believe that eating rare flesh or nearly rare flesh is healthier because the blood-filled meat implies freshness, and fresher meat means more vitamins, protein, and minerals. This is absolutely foolish to think. The Honorable Elijah Muhammad warns us against consuming the blood of any animal.

Although cooked vegetables are best for health, this benefit is dependent on the type of vegetables eaten. In some cases, it matters not whether a vegetable is cooked or raw, the vegetable remains poisonous. Cooking food not only makes the food palatable, but it should also destroy the poisons contained in it. However, some foods contain poisons that are stable against normal cooking. The vegetables that the Honorable Elijah Muhammad deemed unfit for human consumption are stable against heat, and therefore, remain poisonous when ingested. The various poisons contained in most vegetables are described in the book, *Nuts Are Not Good For Humans: Consequences of Human Consumption*, written by this author.

3

Proper Time to Eat

Why does the Honorable Elijah Muhammad state that we must eat no more than one meal every 24 hours?

When we speak of eating once a day, meaning one meal every 24 hours, we are referring to the concept of "meal-time frequency". This is the most overlooked aspect of diet, and is at the core of the great deception perpetrated by this world's food and health industries. Why do I state this? Because careful attention to this area represents the greatest threat to these profit centers; therefore, you will find little mentioned about this subject in mainstream dietary and nutritional recommendations.

Furthermore, few scientific studies are conducted to determine the benefits or detriments associated with "meal-time frequencies". Current research has focused on dietary restriction, a concept that suggests that eating less food retards aging; and caloric restriction, which hypothesizes that consuming fewer calories, will retard aging and improve health. Studies have shown benefits in both dietary approaches; however, both fall extremely short of the goal of substantially increasing human lifespan.

Through the years, the government and public health institutions have rendered bogus dietary recommendations, which have influenced people to eat 3 and 4 meals a day. For years, the proverbial verbiage was "you gotta have your three squares". This anthem came through the mouths of doctors, who at that time, were not required to know much about nutrition. They were merely advising their patients from broadly accepted concepts, and not from scientific fact. The "3-square meal" concept was constantly repeated to the point that it became accepted as a medical truth.

There was never any true scientific research that justified the eating three meals a day. No evidence exists today. The dietary advice to eat three meals a day—breakfast, lunch and dinner—is driven by food, medical and drug industries for profit's sake. They raked in trillions of dollars through bogus advice.

Before answering this question, let us define the term *meal*. According to some dictionaries, *"a meal is the functional unit of eating or is a discrete bout of eating, and has three phases—initiation, maintenance, and termination.* When we eat a meal, there is a beginning and ending to it. Usually, dinner begins with soup and ends with dessert. The main course is served between these two. This discrete bout of eating can last two or more hours.

An important consideration with respect to this issue is that of snacking. Is a snack a meal? Snacks may not be as bodacious as a 4-course meal, but eating them represents a discrete eating bout. So, in truth, there is no such thing as snacking—in that snacking places less of a burden on the digestive system than does a meal. It does not.

When meals and snacks are added together throughout the day, a meal can last all day, which is extremely harmful. We may call our eating segments breakfast, lunch and dinner, but if it mirrors the same eating pattern as hogs in troths, then unless hogs are distinctly fed breakfast, lunch and dinner, we cannot truly apply these terms to our eating habits.

Now, in answering this question of why we should not eat more than one meal every 24 hours, we will briefly describe the digestive process with respect to the time it takes to digest a meal. We will then consider the on-going research about the body's biological clock, which is based on a 24-hour cycle. This research bears witness to certain truths about diet, as given by the Honorable Elijah Muhammad.

The human digestion process is a monumental event, requiring 24 or more hours to completely digest a meal. Depending on the quality of the food, it takes the stomach approximately 4 hours to work on the food, making it suitable to pass to the small intestine.[1] This is the gastric phase of digestion.

In this phase, the food is turned into a liquidly substance called *chyme*. The chyme is gradually released through a small channel (pyloric sphincter) that leads to the small intestine. This process is regulated to avoid an overflow of chyme into the small intestine; thus only small amounts enter at a time.

---

1.   Elaine N. Marieb RN, Ph.D. Human Anatomy and Physiology. Third ed. Redwood, CA: The Benjamin/ Cummings Publishing Company, Inc., 1995.

Here, we ask this question: *What happens when more food is eaten during this process?* For example, if you ate food at noon, how then does the body respond when more food is eaten 2 hours later, while the food is yet in the gastric phase? We can safely assume that the current digestive activity is disturbed. This consideration goes deeper in that although people may think they are hungry at 2 o'clock, the food they ate at noon is still in the digestive process. *How then could their bodies really be calling for food?* Their bodies are not calling for food. This is all in their heads. This point is covered in Question 6.

While in the small intestine many digestive enzymes work on chyme—the enzymes native to the small intestine and the enzymes delivered from the pancreas and the liver (bile) into the small intestine. This is where the nutrients are severed into basic units. Only basic units, such as amino acids (protein) and monosaccharides (carbohydrates) are permitted to pass through the small intestine into the bloodstream. This, of course, is only when the small intestine is functioning properly.

When the organ is malfunctioning, larger molecules and other substances can permeate it and enter the bloodstream. To some extent, the small intestine acts as a filter because large molecules such as whole proteins are denied absorption through the organ. It takes approximately 8 hours to degrade the nutrients, and pass them through intestines into the bloodstream.

We can ask the same question previously asked: *What happens when a person eats more food, adding it to the food they ate several hours earlier, which is still in the digestive process?* Again, how could any person justify hunger at 6 o'clock when the food they ate at noon is still in the digestive process? They cannot. Think on this.

The indigestible material passes to the large intestine or colon. There, some minerals and vitamins, and water are absorbed. The waste matter passes to the rectum for elimination. The large intestine requires approximately 12 hours to complete its digestive functions.

Ideally, it takes approximately 24 hours to properly process a meal—from ingestion to elimination. The Honorable Elijah Muhammad states that some foods take 36 hours to digest.[2] There, however, is still the issue of the time it takes to disseminate the nutrients to the body cells. After the nutrients—amino acids, fats, and carbohydrates—are absorbed through the small intestine, they go to the liver, and then assimilate through the bloodstream where the body cells receive them. *How long does this process take?*

In addition to this primary point, which is that we are only justified in eating one meal every 24 hours, another issue is that we should eat nutritional meals and not snacks because snacks will not provide the nutrients required, yet they will tie up the digestive process. The Honorable Elijah Muhammad advises that we not snack. An adult should eat one meal, and allow it time to serve the body's needs. Eating more food while a meal is not fully digested taxes the digestive organs and compromises the digestion of the food already in the process. Now let us consider research that also proves the Honorable Elijah Muhammad correct.

Since the mid-1900's, scientists have been studying biological cycles in several different organisms. By the 1960's, they had learned that these biological cycles or *circadian rhythms* were generated internally and synchronized to the 24-hour day. The word "circadian" means "around a day". A rhythm is a sequence of events that repeat themselves in time, in the same order and with the same interval. Thus, a circadian rhythm is a biological event or function that repeats through time and in the same order, which is within or about the 24-hour cycle.

These circadian rhythms are consistent with environmental cycles or rhythms that the Earth's rotation dictates. The Honorable Elijah Muhammad teaches that it takes the Earth 23 hours, 56 minutes, and 46 seconds to complete a cycle around its axis. Scientists believe that the Earth's cycle also dictates the body's biological activities. They further believe that these rhythms, when interrupted or disharmonious, cause illness, disease, and premature death.

Scientists believe that nearly all organisms—bacteria, plants, and mammals—have biological clocks, which govern these rhythms. For example, the biological clocks in birds are located in the pineal gland or in the hypothalamus. In some insects, this clock is located in the retina of the eye. In humans, medical scientists have suggested that this clock resides in the hypothalamus. This clock is also called the *suprachiasmatic nuclei* (SCN).

---

2. Muhammad E. Do Not Eat Between Meals. How To Eat To Live. Vol. 2. Chicago: Muhammad's Temple of Islam No. 2, 1972;39.

Circadian rhythms regulate biological processes such as sleep, body temperature, hormone production and digestion. We have already shown that digestion of a meal takes approximately 24 hours. Studies conducted with lower animals confirmed this. For example, one experiment showed that rats anticipated feedings when fed once a day within a window around 24 hours, such as every 23 hours, every 24 hours, and every 27 hours.

Through these experiments, scientists discovered that limiting food access to a particular time of day had profound effects on the behavior and physiology of animals. They have termed this specific behavior *pre-meal behavioral activation*. Physiological activities such as a rise in core temperature, elevated serum corticosterone, and an increase in duodenal (small intestine) disaccharides were observed in rats as their scheduled feeding approached and they anticipated this feeding.

However, the rats lost the ability to anticipate scheduled feedings when the feedings occurred outside that window, such as every 21 hours or every 30 hours. These events confirmed the existence of an internal clock controlling the rats' ability to anticipate a feeding.

A second set of experiments showed that, like any phenomenon governed by a clock, the rats could not adjust in one cycle when feeding schedules shifted by a large amount of time. When feeding schedules shifted by 8 hours, it took two to five cycles for the rats to anticipate feedings at the new time.

Two other experiments conducted in the late 1970s by Dr. Frederick Stephan, a neuroscientist at Florida State University and founder of the SCN in the human brain, showed that digestion was not entirely governed by the SCN. The first study showed that rats fed only once a day anticipated their feedings one to three hours ahead of time. Again, this confirmed that a biological clock was influencing their feeding behavior. The scientists assumed that the SCN governed this.

However, in another feeding study, the SCN was destroyed, and the rats continued to behave according to their set feeding patterns. This, of course, confirmed the possible presence of another biological clock that was independent of the SCN, and specifically regulated feeding behaviors. This biological clock has been termed "feeding entrainable oscillator" (FEO).[3] These feeding behaviors are called "gastro-rhythms". An oscillator is a mechanism that allows a steady, uninterrupted rhythm.

This concept, "entrainable oscillator", asserts that a biological clock exists that dictates the call for food. This oscillator, because it is adjustable, gives a mammal power over hunger or the call for food. A gastro-rhythm is evidence that this oscillator makes the call for food at a specific time based on that mammal's trained behavior patterns.

These experiments also revealed the consequence associated with eating when hunger is not present. For example, in studies wherein rats ate ad lib (anytime), they experienced digestive disorders and disease. The scientists noted that such studies provide insight into the epidemic of digestive disorders facing this nation. They specifically pointed to the digestive disorders among the workforce caused by eating lunch and eating that lunch too fast. They questioned whether most people in the workforce are truly hungry when eating lunch, or are merely following a cultural norm. This point is discussed in Question 6.

Just a side note about the use of lower creatures in experiments destined to impact human life via health or nutrition policies. In most circumstances, I frown upon such experiments for obvious reasons. Lower creatures do not reflect the total spectrum of human life—biologically, behaviorally, or otherwise. However, the Honorable Elijah Muhammad states that all creatures maintain their lives through diet, and that certain animals have short lifespans because they eat anything and eat all day. Reasonably, a regulated diet should benefit most, if not all, animals. Their experiments, therefore, have merit.

These studies are very significant in that they confirm that feeding behavior patterns are adjustable because the biological mechanism that dictates this behavior is trainable. Again, this validates these words from the Honorable Elijah Muhammad:[4]

> *Within one week you can get used to eating once a day, and within one week you can get used to eating once every other day. Many of the Muslims are eating like this, and you can eat this way too. Our stomachs are just the way we train them to be.*

At present, scientists are trying to find the location of this FEO, as well as what cues it, and how it signals the brain to change the behavior of the

---

3.   Stephan FK. The "Other" Circadian System: Food as a Zeitgeber. Journal of Biological Rhythms 2002;17(4):284-292(9).

4.   Muhammad, E., How To Eat To Live. Vol. 1. 1967, Chicago, IL: Final Call Publishing Company. 24-25

organism. Scientists speculate that the cells that make up this clock are located somewhere in the liver. I have reservations about this specific notion. My position, when it comes to humans, is that our brain dictates all behavior. This is where obscurities in science can develop, as some scientists attempt to fit the physiological and neurological workings of lower creatures into those of humans. They should be very cautious about this. Humans are governed by intelligence and not instinct, per se.

Whether scientists discover this FEO is not as important as the critical truths proven by this research. One truth is that the best diet for humans is one that includes partaking of food at 24-hour regulated periods. Another truth is that we have power to train our bodies to call for food when we want them to call for food. This means that we can govern our eating behavior to support the best diet for humans. Biologically, such a diet includes eating one meal every 24 hours. This is the proper time to eat.

4

Between 4 - 6 p.m.

Why did the Honorable Elijah Muhammad suggest that the best the time to eat is between the hours of 4 and 6 p.m.?

The primary emphasis in *How To Eat To Live* is that we eat no more than one meal every 24 hours. Whether that meal is eaten at noon or 3 p.m.— we are strongly advised to eat at the same hour the next day. The Honorable Elijah Muhammad also expressed that the timeframe of 4 to 6 p.m. is the best time to eat.[1]

What first comes to mind when considering this recommendation is the question about breakfast—*what about this being the most important meal?* Breakfast is an important meal for the merchants who run the food industry, but there is no proof that it is the most important meal for humans, unless you are eating your one-meal-a-day in the morning. However, this is not the case with most people. Breakfast launches the destructive *three-meals-a-day* run. More can be stated about this "breakfast" ploy, and how we have been duped into following something that has no scientific basis.

If the ideal time to eat is between the hours of 4 and 6 p.m., then it would hold that neither breakfast nor lunch hours are appropriate times for humans to intake food. Let us view one of several reasons why this is so.

Previously, we discussed circadian rhythms and learned that through our biological clocks, processes such as sleep, body temperature, hormone production and digestion are regulated, and that this regulation is based on the Earth's 24-hour rotation around its axis. We now examine one area of hormone production regulation that gives insight into why the best time to eat is later in the afternoon and not in the morning.

---

1. Muhammad E. The Proper Food and The Proper Time to Eat It. How To Eat To Live, Book 1. Vol. 1. Chicago, IL: Final Call Publishing Company, 1967;32

Various hormones participate in the digestive process. Some hormones signal organs to release digestive enzymes into the stomach and small intestine, while others control the provision of nutrients by releasing them into the bloodstream. One such hormone that has the role of the latter function is cortisol.

Cortisol is the most potent glucocorticoid produced by the adrenal gland. The adrenal gland or suprarenal gland is one of several endocrine glands. It is about 2 in. (5.1 cm) long and is situated atop each kidney. The outer layer of the adrenal gland secretes about 30 steroid hormones, with aldosterone and cortisol considered the most important.

Figure 1. Adrenal Gland (atop kidney)

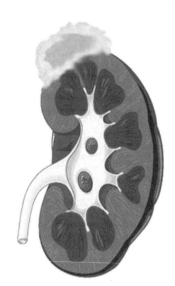

Cortisol is synthesized from cholesterol and its production, as with all hormones, is regulated through a biofeedback mechanism. Cortisol is released when the pituitary gland releases the adrenocorticotropic hormone (ACTH). Release of this hormone is regulated by corticotropin releasing factor (CRF). CRF travels through the hypothalamo-pituitary portal vessels to the anterior pituitary gland, where it stimulates release of ACTH. ACTH then travels in the bloodstream to the adrenal cortex, where cortisol is produced in response to ACTH stimulation. Approximately 20 milligrams of cortisol are secreted by the adrenal cortex each day.

Cortisol acts through specific intracellular receptors and affects numerous physiologic systems including immune function, glucose counter regulation, vascular tone, and bone metabolism. The normal function of cortisol is to help the body respond to stress and change. It mobilizes nutrients, modifies the body's response to inflammation, stimulates the liver to raise the blood sugar, and it helps control the amount of water in the body. The metabolic functions of cortisol are:

- Increases plasma levels of amino acids, fatty acids, glucose, and glycerol.
- Stimulates uptake of amino acids by the liver and subsequent gluconeogenesis. Free cortisol binds to hepatocytes and stimulates RNA polymerase to produce more RNA, which in turn synthesizes more proteins. The enzymes then begin converting pyruvate to glucose-6-phosphate and metabolizing amino acids (TYR, GLY, and TRP). Amino acids are deaminated and converted into glucose.
- Lowers the levels of phosphodiesterase, increasing cAMP, which plays a role in gluconeogenesis.
- Increases return of free glucose to the blood at the end of the gluconeogenetic pathway.
- Inhibits glucose uptake by muscle and adipose tissue.
- Has permissive action on the ability of epinephrine and growth hormone to cause lipolysis in adipose tissue.
- Besides increasing glucose metabolism, cortisol also enhances the arteriole contractive response to norepinephrine, inhibits arteriole dilation, closes capillary sphincters, and causes the heart to contract more strongly, allowing glucose to be directed to tissues that need it most (the brain).

ACTH and cortisol are secreted according to a 24-hour circadian rhythm, with a peak secretion early in the morning and a nadir late at night. Figures 2 and 3 show the circadian rhythm of ACTH and cortisol.

This daily rhythm persists regardless of food intake and sleep/wake cycles. Although certain factors may cause an increase in cortisol levels, the basic rhythm continues. The anterior pituitary and adrenal gland are more sensitive to CRF and ACTH, respectively, at the peak of the rhythm.

The degree of corticotropic stress response is highest at the nadir of the circadian rhythm.

Figure 2. Cortisol Secretion[2]

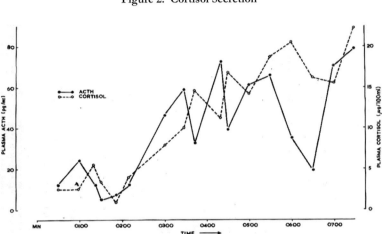

Stress can cause stimulation of the hypothalamus, which releases CRH. This can cause an excess of cortisol in the bloodstream. There are several diseases linked to excess cortisol secretion and such diseases are considered stress-related or stress-induced.

As noted, one of the metabolic roles of cortisol is to increase plasma levels of amino acids, fatty acids, glucose, and glycerol.[3] This is precisely what occurs when a person eats food. The body is provided the nutrients required to energize and sustain it. So, in essence, the nutrients we seek to obtain from food are already provided.

Cortisol begins acting before we arise from sleep because it has a key role in ensuring that the energy required to get us up and going is provided. If this did not occur, we would not have the energy to awaken. Figure 1 shows that cortisol is heavily secreted between the hours of 3 and 8 a.m. Figure 2

2.   Daily Rhythm of Cortisol Secretion. Vol. 2002 University of Arkansas, Faytetteville; http://comp.uark.edu/ ~gmh01/cortisol2.html#Cortisol%20Transport

3.   Hucklebridge FH, Clow A, Abeyguneratne T, Huezo-Diaz P, Evans P. The Awakening Cortisol Response and Blood Glucose Levels. Life Sciences 1999;64(11):931-937.

shows cortisol secretion over a 24-hour period. As shown, cortisol continues its peak secretion beyond noon. Again, this calls into question the need for lunch, as well as breakfast.

Figure 3. Cortisol Secretion in 24-h period[4]

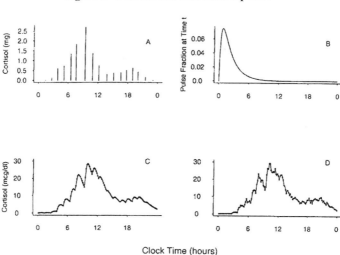

Clock Time (hours)

Observing cortisol from a different view, its action releases those nutrients that are already stored or circulating in the body. This gives us another view of digestion. Obviously, the meal eaten the previous day must produce some benefit for us the following morning. This is precisely the case, given the fact that the nutrients are likely being assimilated at that time of the morning. Albeit, the body contains the nutrients necessary to get us going in the morning without our having to consume more food, which makes our having to eat both meals unnecessary.

We can now see that this hormone is responsible for initiating major metabolic activities on our behalf. Our Creator has innately factored in those biological processes required for us to arise from deep sleep, and get through most of the day.

4.   Brown EN, Meehan PM, Dempster AP. A stochastic differential equation model of diurnal cortisol patterns. American Journal of Physiology Endocrinology and Metabolism 2001;280(3):E450-E461.

We must also continue to keep in the mind the digestive process covered in Question 3. Digestion is a 24-hour process, so if we ate dinner at 6 p.m., why do we need to eat breakfast the next morning? We do not. We already possess enough nutrients to function adequately the next morning. These biological workings transcend our personal opinions and even the discomfort we might experience by not eating "our breakfast".

We have the greater right to modify our behaviors based on scientific truths rather than continue to follow lies or obey our urges and emotions. We must keep in mind that humans are governed by intelligence, and any lack of it, or rejection of the truth that proceeds from it, places us in harms way.

Our personal experience provides additional support to aid our understanding of the biological processes governed by cortisol secretion. Most of us have experienced tiredness or fatigue when attempting to rise in the morning after eating late at night. Remember, the circadian rhythm that regulates cortisol is independent of other biological mechanisms including digestion. Therefore, the late night meal or snack places a terrific burden on the body because digestion is one of the most demanding biological activities the body engages. The body is now overwhelmed with the major tasks employed through cortisol and the digestive tasks resulting from the late night meal or snack.

We should ask ourselves: *What happens when we add a meal to the provision of nutrients already in process through cortisol action?* This directly addresses the "breakfast" issue. Each of us can testify to the conditions that ensue after eating breakfast. If honest, we would admit that eating breakfast clouds the thinking, and the body becomes fatigued under the burden of digestion.

This, primarily, refers to adults and not children. The nutritional requirements that support body growth are different from those required to sustain the body. Children require two meals, which could include breakfast, as they are still growing. Adults may require an additional meal, which could include breakfast, if they are ill. The Honorable Elijah Muhammad has stated that a person may need to eat more than once a day to fight illness.

On a side note, adults are so eager to boast maturity in that we have put away *childish things* due to our maturity. We proudly quote the Biblical passage *"when I was a child, I thought as a child; but now that I am a man, I have put away childish things"*. Well, how about this: *when I was a child, I ate as a child; now that I am an adult, I have put away the childish way of eating.* Because people continue to eat as children, they are sent to the grave very early.

In this circadian process, specifically as we approach evening hours, which is congruent with the "setting of the Sun", and the lowering of energy levels, eating becomes necessary. During this period, cortisol levels drop significantly so the provision of nutrients afforded through cortisol action decreases. The chart shown in Figure 3 demonstrates this, as cortisol secretion dives significantly. Therefore, we may require food in the late afternoon to raise our energy levels. This is why the timeframe between 4 and 6 p.m. is the ideal time to eat.

Eating at this time not only replenishes our bodies, but we are doing it in a timeframe that is still within the "active" day. In short, we are not eating so late that we do not have the time to engage in some physical activity to aid digestion. We are not eating so late that we are sleeping on a load of food.

Some health scientists have suggested that a short walk after dinner aids digestion, making it easy for us to rest properly later that night. If we assume that most people turn in at 9 or 10 p.m., then eating at 6 p.m. allows us nearly 3 to 4 hours of activity. This is enough time to get us nearly through the gastric phase of digestion. This is wise.

Our lives should be lived in comfort, which is achievable through the biological processes that support life and longevity. The Honorable Elijah Muhammad has truly provided a new paradigm for health and longevity.

5

Methuselah

Why does the first sentence of the first chapter in How To Eat To Live (Book 2) mention Methuselah?

The Honorable Elijah Muhammad writes:

Eat to live to bring about a return to perfection and long life, like Noah and Methuselah, who lived nearly 1000 years of our calendar year (containing 365 1/4 days).

Following are words of caution concerning our perception about the above quotation. Although some people are prone to take these words by the Honorable Elijah Muhammad as a jest, these words provide the solution to the on-going quest of the scientific community to discover the "fountain of youth". We should not think trivial about the divine guidance of the Honorable Elijah Muhammad, especially the power contained in it to establish the new and everlasting paradigm for human longevity.

Additionally, we should be mindful that there is nearly six billion people on the planet and that many circles for the acquisition of knowledge exist. The smallest to the largest creatures are being studied. The Sun, as well as the smallest stars, is being studied. Human potential in every conceivable way, including longevity, is also being intensely studied.

In the quest to learn the ways to extend human life, scientists target the great patriarch, Methuselah, because his is the longest age recorded—969 years. So, simply stated, by mentioning Methuselah in *How To Eat To Live*, the Honorable Elijah Muhammad is informing all—the average *Joe* and the so-called scientist—that He possesses the knowledge to increase human life into the hundreds of years.

The average person might find this of little interest or value. However, scientists have viewed such knowledge as very valuable. Here, lies the difference between the learned and the unlearned when it comes to serious matters of life.

The masses are generally unaware of the discussions, research, and scientific studies engaged to determine the upper limits of human lifespans. The poor quality of life, particularly of health, experienced by the majority is proof that gross negligence exists about matters concerning life extension. This is because most people are trained to live for the moment—recklessly seeking to satisfy our urges for food, sex, security, and pleasure, while planning to retire from the workforce and die around the age of 65 years. The former ensures the later, so even those who meticulously plan for their retirement through 401(k)s and other money-saving vehicles are not considered super intelligent.

In the end, this pool of "saved" money will quickly dissipate through healthcare costs, as is currently happening at a phenomenal rate to millions of people. How are people justified in saving money for their alleged "senior" years, but not seek to preserve their youthfulness and health to stave off the ill-health that usually accompanies those "senior" years? This is not intelligent. Intelligence, in this case, is to know Almighty God's expectation for our lives, including life expectancy, and seek the truths that enable us to fulfill His expectations.

After knowing Almighty God's expectations for our lives, we can build our personal expectations around His expectations. One of Almighty God's expectations is, in fact, to extend human lifespan. The Scriptures teach that when the Messiah comes He will give us life, and more life abundantly. If this is true, then He must set an expectation, as well as acquaint us with our potential to live into the hundreds of years. He has done both through the guidance given to us by the Honorable Elijah Muhammad and through the words He shared with the Honorable Elijah Muhammad about His personal expectation for long life.

For example, the Honorable Elijah Muhammad shared with us that His Teacher, Allah in Person; Master Fard Muhammad would live a minimum of one year for every year that we (Black People of America) were enslaved in America. This is 400 years. He did not tell us the maximum number of years that He would live, but we know that He has the power to live longer than 400 years. We expect Almighty God to possess such power.

Of course, many of us (Muslims) use this as a conversation piece to boast the power of Almighty God, but in this information, we find valuable principles. One principle is that we, as humans, have the power to set expectations for our lives, including the number of years we would like to enjoy life. Another principle is that we should set this expectation or goal.

There is power in setting an expectation to live a certain number of years. Let us look carefully into this.

Who among us desires to live only 65 years? We can safely assume that few people only want 65 years of life, even though they may plan their retirement for age 65. On another note, we should be cautioned in subscribing to this "retirement" concept. Because, despite the fact that we may not readily declare our desire to live until age 65, are we not subversively declaring such in our retirement planning? After all, is not retirement synonymous with *"I'll be dead shortly after I retire"*? These concepts are Satan's way of subtly forming our minds for self-destruction and premature death.

We declare our expectations to get married, to attend college, and to have specific careers. We declare our expectations for many things. However, how many of us state a desire to live a certain length of time, such as 100, 125, or 150 years? What could a person accomplish in 100 years that he or she cannot accomplish in 65 years? Of course, with more time, we can accomplish more things and help more people. Dr. Martin Luther King, Jr. stated, "Longevity has its place".[1] It does. One document states the following about the value of long lifespans:[2]

> Long life spans, they point out, offer numerous advantages to humans and other animals that live in social communities rather than individually. Small increases in longevity can be amplified in successive generations, leading to even greater longevity.
>
> For example, a longer life allows more opportunity for humans and other species over time to develop the biological mechanisms that at older ages will maintain health and repair physical flaws. Increased longevity also makes it possible for older individuals to nurture and pass on resources to the younger generation.
>
> And, as the life span lengthens and experience increases efficiency, the products of the labor of the community can be reinvested among several generations, allowing individuals to specialize in their areas of strength, fostering innovations that, in turn, promote longer life.

---

1. Dr. Martin Luther King J. Speech given in Memphis, Tennessee to help the sanitation workers who were on strike., April 3, 1968.
2. Lengthy lifespans may have evolutionary link. Vol. 2002 Dateline UC Davis, University of California, Davis, 2001.

Much can be stated about each benefit given above. For example, the most natural and effective way to produce a healthier population is to consistently increase the wellness of that population generation-after-generation. This has always been the natural order of things. Man is perfected by way of constancy and time. This is, however, contingent upon submission to the right guidance. Submitting to the wrong dietary guidance will only maintain a legacy of poor health. This is the precise problem afflicting the human family, the world over.

If each generation maintains the same destructive behavior as the previous generation, then improvement is not possible. In driving this point further, consider the disastrous health plight faced by Black people in America. This crisis is largely due to stubbornness, and rejection of a better way of life. Too many of us continue to eat bad food—ham hocks, kale, pig feet, sweet potatoes, and an array of grease-laden foods; and drink beer, wine, and whiskey. As a result, our health condition continues to worsen, generation-after-generation. This behavior, by each generation, places the following generation at risk, and robs them of an increase in their potential to improve the overall quality of life.

On the other hand, as we submit to proper dietary guidance and a righteous way of life, each generation will live longer than the previous generation. Each generation will advance civilization. We will be a more productive people. Research has already proven this.[3] This is not only for Black people, but also for all people.

The populace, however, is being duped by the "genetic engineering" debacle. The selfish quest of this world's scientists to go directly to the human genome for life extension, but not change destructive behavior patterns, is quickly proving futile. Allah willing, this area will be covered in another FAQ volume.

In contemplating the purpose for knowing Master Fard Muhammad's expectation to live a minimum of one year for every year His people spent in bondage, I believe that we are given this to consider our individual expectations for longer life. A person, also, can declare his or her desire to live 100, 125, or 200 years. Some might think *"Well, its up to Almighty God how long I live."* This is true. It is up to Almighty God if you live

3.   News BBC. No 'limit' to human life span. BBC News, 2000.

tomorrow; however, your behavior also has something to do with whether you live or die tomorrow. The Creator did not give us a free will and hold back our ability for self-determination. This is part of the free will. We are free to choose and act as we determine.

For example, if a person gobbled down fatty foods for 30 years of his or her life, and as a result developed clogged arteries, then when heart failure occurred, he or she could not get away with stating that the *"the Lord willed this"*. This is nonsense. That person chose to eat this way. That person determined to eat grease-laden food, and Almighty God did not interfere with that determination.

Now, we can agree that Almighty God's Permissive Will allowed that person to go into heart failure, but His Active Will was not involved in it. His Permissive Will, to an extent, is the natural consequences of our own actions. His Permissive Will is also in the natural laws He setup to govern life. The process of sowing and reaping is a natural law. If we sow good, we reap good. On the other hand, if we sow wrong, we reap the consequences of that wrong. Understanding these natural laws is just as important as understanding Almighty God.

Certainly, Almighty God has the power to intervene in any health situation, but the greatest of His interventions is guidance and an example through a servant He raises from among the people to teach them how to think and act, which includes how to eat to live. Therefore, why should anyone expect Almighty God to intervene in the destructive consequences of rebellion against that which He has already supplied as an intervention? In many cases, we are left to suffer the painful consequences for rejecting the truth. Now back to the life expectancy subject.

We have the natural and innate ability to "desire" things for ourselves. If we desire a financial nest egg to help us through retirement, then why should we not desire a longer stay on the earth? If Almighty God, through our ability to learn, enables us to develop the methods by which we can build a nest egg, then cannot the same be done to help us achieve longer life? Of course! We only need that knowledge which will help us achieve this. The desire, however, must be present.

Without the desire to live long, we are prone to lack the conscientiousness about the most critical activities that support life—our thoughts and food. The result of not having this desire or goal is gross negligence. A reckless, error-prone existence is the consequence. Many people are currently living such a life.

Now, suppose you declared that you wanted to live 150 years. You now must determine, and then assess, those factors associated with reaching this goal. Certainly, you could not continue a lifestyle that takes you down by age 60, because the result would be death by age 60. By lifestyle, we mean how one behaves. This includes what we eat and how often we eat it. There are other factors that must be controlled to live long; however, our focus in this context is diet.

So, a person could not continue to eat as did those who lived only 60 or so years, and expect to live 150 years. That person would have to follow dietary guidance that enables a person to live 150 or so years. This, of course, is a deeply rich subject. Allah willing, we will go further in another volume. But, suffice it to say that, those seeking a diet that will permit them to live 150 years must know where to find it. Where does one look?

The most obvious, yet perhaps the most overlooked, place to look is in books. The seeker must find those diet books wherein the authors have made such a claim—that practicing the diet or diets touted in the respective book will help a person live 150 years or longer. This approach is extremely prudent, particularly when there are hundreds, if not thousands, of diet books available. The goal to live 150 years serves as a filter, so those diet books or pamphlets that omit longevity goals or claims are immediately tossed aside.

In the end, only a few books will make the cut on the claim alone. Those books not making the cut will include the voluminous health encyclopedias, and nutrition and diet books that describe every disease, herb, and element known, but never delineate how these things work together to promote longevity.

To further siphon the remaining books, the next task of the person seeking to live 150 years is to examine the dietary prescriptions and pit them against the longevity claims made in the books. By dietary prescription, we mean the precise and complete dietary instructions.

A prescription is defined as: *1) the act of establishing official rules, laws, or directions; and 2) a written order, especially by a physician, for the preparation and administration of a medicine or other treatment.* A dietary prescription must identify the foods to eat, how these foods should be prepared, and the best time to eat these foods. These core factors support longevity, but only when such a prescription is based on science, specifically those sciences that relate to the human body, with emphasis on the digestion process. This is how medication is assessed and prescribed. Therefore, if diet is the best preventive medicine, then we should be no less meticulous about prescribing the right diet than we are about prescribing the right medication.

Many books promote diets that only tell a person what to eat, but not how to prepare the food and when to eat it. Such diets fail to meet the criteria necessary to classify them as dietary prescriptions, so they should be tossed into the pile with the other inadequate materials.

Now, how should we assess a dietary prescription's capacity to produce longer life? Let us view longevity from the perspective of safety. If we are safe from injury and harm, then our chances to live long are increased. Injury, in any form, contains the potential to end life. Therefore, a dietary prescription must ensure safety of the body. It must not injure the person.

The Honorable Elijah Muhammad repeatedly states this point throughout *How To Eat To Live—how to keep food from hurting us.* Food can injure us if it is not the proper food. It can also injure us if the food is not prepared correctly. It can injure us if it is eaten too often. These injuries are against the organs that regulate or support digestion. Injury to these organs disrupts the metabolic processes that support life.

Therefore, an adequate dietary prescription must be in harmony with these biological and metabolic processes. It must work for them and not against them. To my knowledge, *How To Eat To Live (books 1 & 2)* is the only diet that contains the dietary prescription that caters to these essentials; thereby promoting longevity, as defined by Almighty God, which has an upper limit of 1,000 years. Methuselah nearly made it there, only falling 31 years short.

6

Eating Before We Are Hungry

*Why does the Honorable Elijah Muhammad state that 95%
of our sickness comes from eating before we are hungry?*

Careful thought would lead us to assume that when food is put in the body before the body calls for it, this food is not properly digested. The Honorable Elijah Muhammad confirms this throughout *How To Eat To Live*, supporting our assumptions.

Poor digestion can lead to illness. Therefore, we can safely assume that putting one's digestive system to work before it calls for food and is prepared to receive food, causes illness. In light of this assumption, this "call" for food creates the best environment for proper digestion. In this, two things must be determined, biologically. We must first determine what constitutes true hunger. By true hunger, we mean the real call of the body for nutrition and not merely the symptoms that we assume to be the call for food. One symptom is the growling of the stomach. There are also other symptoms.

The second issue that must be determined is the preparedness of the body to receive food when true hunger is present, as opposed to when it is not. This issue goes to the core of how illness is caused when the body is not prepared to receive food.

Before proceeding, we must reinforce the foundational premise of *How To Eat To Live*, which is that humans (adults) should eat no more than one meal every 24 hours. This premise, which is the basis of the dietary law of God, was addressed and substantiated in Question 3. Now, let us consider "true" hunger.

How do we know when we are hungry, especially given the fact that we can experience symptoms of hunger often throughout any given day? Many theories have been issued to explain the biological mechanisms that cause the feeling of hunger. These include the *stomach contraction*, *glucose*, *insulin*, *fatty acid*, and the *heat-production* theories.[1]

The *stomach contraction* theory states that we know we are hungry when our stomach contracts.[2] This is the symptom of growling, which we will cover in detail because most people believe that they are hungry when their stomachs growl. The *glucose* theory states that we feel hungry when our blood glucose level is low,[3] which drives us to eat. The *insulin* theory states that we feel hungry when our insulin level increases suddenly in our bodies.[4] The *fatty acid* theory states that our bodies have receptors that detect an increase in the level of fatty acid,[5] and the activation of the receptor for fatty acids triggers hunger. The *heat-production* theory states that we feel hungry when our body temperature drops, and when it rises again, the hunger decreases.[6] These theories have been tested, causing some to be outright refuted by research, and wisely so, because some of them are illogical. Now let us tackle the issue of growling.

Following is an excellent explanation about the biological cause of "growling":[7]

> The growling of your stomach (and intestines too) has to do with the presence of air within your gut. Your gut is a hollow tube that is lined with muscle. This muscle contracts even when you are hungry, producing waves of activity known as Migrating Myoelectric Complexes. The term 'myoelectric' has to do with the electrical activity of contracting muscle (myo=muscle).
>
> Between meals these Migrating Myoelectric Complexes propagate along the entire length of the gut. The continued contractions of the stomach and intestines serve to keep mucus, remaining foodstuffs and bacteria from accumulating at any one site. The contractions also produce vibrations when air bubbles become trapped in the lumen. These vibrations produce the growling noises associated with hunger.

In this explanation, growling is the reaction of that which is done to detoxify and maintain the stomach. Here is another good explanation of growling:[8]

1. Hara T. Hunger and Eating. Vol. 2002 California State University, Northridge, 1997
2. Coon, D. (1995). Introduction to Psychology: Exploration and Application, 7th ed. MN:West Publishing Company
3. Franken, R. E. (1994). Human Motivation, 3rd ed. CA: Brooks/Cole Publishing Company.
4. Heller, R. F., & Heller, R. F. (1991). The Carbohydrate Addict's Diet. New York: Penguin Books USA Inc.

Stomach growling occurs when the stomach receives signals to begin digestion but the stomach is empty; the motion of the stomach muscles begins, but the organ is hollow. The obvious solution is to eat, but this is not always practical.

That which is obvious is only obvious until knowledge comes to pull the mask off the obvious, making it otherwise. As stated, most believe that growling is a sign of hunger. Now that we know that adults should only eat one meal every 24 hours, when growling occurs a few hours after we eat, we are forced to see this physiological phenomenon as something other than a true call for food. Eating food when growling occurs is impractical. It disrupts our dietary regimen, that is, if we have achieved regularity to our diets.

We have the power to determine how our bodies respond, but this is best achieved through regulation. The Honorable Elijah Muhammad states that we must have regularity to everything we do. If we react to every growl by eating, we will never gain regularity to our diets and we will never get the growling under control. By following the dietary guidance in *How To Eat To Live*, we gain complete control over our bodies.

Part of this control rest in our psychological approach to eating, which includes our overall view of food. In short, we have to see food as a means to an end and not merely as a means with no end associated with it. The latter is the prevailing mindset when it comes to how food is viewed. The adage *"eating to be eating"* is the very thing that most people do. This is why many health researchers agree that symptoms of hunger are psychologically triggered, and have little to do with true hunger.

Our learned and cognitive behaviors trigger hunger symptoms. These behaviors can be classified as appetite. These terms 'appetite' and 'hunger' are often used interchangeably, but they are very distinct. In *How To Eat To Live*, the distinction between hunger and appetite is pointed out. In one statement, the Honorable Elijah Muhammad warns us against letting our appetites get us into trouble by consuming food all day and all night. This trouble is sickness, illness, and eventually, death. On several instances, He

5.   Franken, R. E. (1994). Human Motivation, 3rd ed. CA: Brooks/Cole Publishing Company.
6.   Ibid, 1994
7.   Risely, P., Why does my stomach growl? 1996, MadSci Network.
8.   Seitz, P., What causes a stomach to growl and can this be prevented. 1997, National Science Foundation.

states that we should not eat until we are hungry. Therefore, hunger, and not appetite, should dictate our eating habits.

For the sake of distinction, hunger is the physiological need to eat, which is experienced as a drive for obtaining food, and is characterized by an unpleasant sensation that demands relief. This uncomfortable feeling is usually weakness, fatigue or other symptoms of energy deficit. On the other hand, appetite is the psychological desire to eat, which is a learned motivation. This desire is usually triggered by the sight, smell, or thought of appealing foods. Appetite can trigger symptoms of hunger, but we should distinguish true hunger by the intensity and type of the discomfort. Discomfort resulting from appetite is usually confined to growling sensations or something less impressive.

Again, the point with respect to true hunger is that hunger symptoms are not always representative of true hunger. We have learned that by using wisdom to regulate our eating habits to one meal every 24 hours (at a minimum), we can bring hunger symptoms under control and place ourselves in a better position to experience and respond to a true hunger call. Now let us briefly take up the issue of how the body is prepared to receive food.

In the digestive process, gastric secretion is part of that which enables our bodies, or digestive tract, to digest food. Under normal digestive function, gastric secretions amount to approximately 3 liters each day.

This secretion is controlled by neural and hormonal mechanisms. Neural controls are achieved through long and short nerve reflexes. The long nerve reflex is accomplished through the vagus nerve, which is the only cranial nerve that extends beyond the head and neck into the abdomen. The short nerve reflex is facilitated through the enteric nervous system, which is the digestive tract's nervous system.

Gastric secretion is divided into three phases: cephalic, gastric and intestinal. Biochemical and physiological events in the body that are induced by thinking of, smelling, tasting, or chewing food belong to the cephalic phase of digestion. The term *cephalic* has ancient Greek and Latin origins that mean *head*, which implies involvement of the nervous system or the influence of our learned behaviors. The cephalic phase is considered the preparation phase of digestion.

During this phase, the brain gets the stomach ready for digestion. Biologically, inputs from the activated olfactory receptors or taste buds are relayed to the hypothalamus, which in turn stimulates the vagal nuclei of the brain (medulla oblongata), causing motor impulses to be transmitted through the vagus nerves to the stomach. This enhanced secretory activity results when we are aroused by food or need food. However, if we are depressed or have no appetite, this part of the cephalic reflex is subdued.

There is other scientific literature that explains the cephalic phase by presenting its connection to how the body or digestive tract handles hunger. This literature cites that the cephalic phase is prompt into action by:[9] *1) the signals that guide selection of food; 2) the thought, sight or smell of food (as already noted); 3) an increase in hunger brought on by lack of food in the stomach; and 4) the increased hunger during an energy deficit.*

Of course, number 4 is the ideal impetus to trigger the cephalic phase because of two reasons. First, the cephalic phase, no matter how physically influential it is in driving us to eat, only stimulates a fraction of the maximum possible levels of gastric and pancreatic sections. This phase does not produce a rise in the levels of gastrin and cholecystokinin (CCK), which are required for adequate digestion.

The potential of maximum output of these digestive juices occurs in the gastric and intestinal phases. This output is contingent upon the intensity of hunger and the availability of the digestive juices. This is a critical point and leads to the second reason.

When the cephalic phase is triggered because of an energy deficit, we can be assured that the biological preparedness of the body to receive food is present in the gastric and intestinal digestive phases. These dynamics represent the true call, which is assessed according to an assembly of several key factors. These factors are intelligence, the training of the digestive system, and the physiological call for food.

By intelligence, we reiterate the premise of the dietary guidance given by the Honorable Elijah Muhammad—to eat only one meal every 24 hours. This way of eating is commensurable with fasting, which accomplishes several key benefits. Generally, eating this way assures that the food is

---

9.   (Instructor), C.N.D.R.B.M., Regulation of Food Intake. 2002, University of California, Davis Campus

properly digested because the body is given proper rest between meal intervals. In this rest, the digestive juices expended during the digestive process are replenished, and thus, available to properly digest the next meal.

This goes to the heart of *preparedness*. True hunger mobilizes the organs and digestive juices to digest a meal. Of course, the adequate amount of digestive juices must be available. They are not available in the necessary amount when food is constantly consumed, as they are expended in a digestive process that continues all day. Neither are the organs strong enough to deal with another meal, when the meals eaten several hours earlier have burdened them.

This means that, scientifically, there is no justification for us to eat food constantly throughout the day under the auspices that we are hungry. If we do this, we will find ourselves constantly depleted of essential digestive juices, which will lead to improper digestion and the degeneration of the organs.

The issue of "training" takes on significance because the Honorable Elijah Muhammad has stated that our bodies can be trained to call for food once every 24 hours, once every 48 hours, once every 72 hours, or once a week. This sheds an entirely new light on the issue of human potential and adaptability. Hunger is a trained condition, or part of a physiological response to a trained condition (dietary regimen). Hunger is not something that invades the body.

This description or definition of hunger simply means that true hunger can only be assessed in association with the key factors (those given above). When the physiological symptoms occur outside the realm of these principal factors, true hunger is, more than likely, not present. The only other condition, with respect to adults, that true hunger may be present outside these conditions is when a person is ill. The body expends energy to fight sickness and heal itself, so food is usually required more readily than every 24 hours.

Eating when true hunger is not present causes illness because the mobilization of digestive juices and the strength of the digestive organs, acting in the digestive process, do not support the proper digestion of food. Allah Willing, we will go further into this topic in forthcoming volumes.

7

Fasting Cures

The Honorable Elijah Muhammad states that medical scientists know that fasting is the cure for 90 percent of our illnesses. How does fasting cure?

Again, we have another powerful statement,[1] which if practiced, would not only disrupt mainstream America's health empire, which includes the trillions of dollars it generates from a populace that is rarely cured of anything, but the practice of fasting would actually vanquish this empire. Adopting fasting as both a preventive and curative modality would quickly expose mainstream health interventions that feature toxic pills and potions for what they truly are—false, bogus, and senseless practices that have profit as the ultimate objective.

Fasting is the voluntary abstinence from eating food for varying lengths of time. Fasting is synonymous with resting. When we abstain from eating food, we are allowing our bodies' time to rest, and through this rest, the body is able to restore and replenish itself. The organs of the body receive a break from the hard work of digestion. The extra energy gives the body the chance to heal and restore itself. Additionally, fasting burns away the toxic substances contained in the stored energy in the muscles.

The digestive tract is exposed to environmental threats namely bacteria, viruses, parasites, and toxins; and therefore requires the greater support from the immune system. When food is broken down in the small intestine, it travels through the blood to the liver, which is the body's chief purifying organ. The liver breaks down and removes the toxic substances produced by digestion. During fasting, the liver also detoxifies. This is extremely important for the body's health.

The concept of fasting is brought into view, if we consider the physical condition we would find ourselves if we were not able to rest and sleep.

1. Muhammad E. Fasting. How To Eat To Live, Book 1. Vol. 1. Chicago, IL: Final Call Publishing Company, 1967;20

Our normal functions would deteriorate, and eventually we would fall out. This is precisely what the body does while constantly under the burden of digestion—deteriorating over a 20 to 40 year period, then ceasing function at the 65 to 70 year mark.

The rest that we engage through sleep and relaxation is not, particularly, the rest the body needs. Our bodies are a compilation of organs. The digestive process burdens many of these vital organs. Therefore, if these organs are to truly rest, they must have a reprieve from digestive activities. Fasting gives the organs the necessary rest.

Before briefly considering the healing power of fasting, let us review some of its history. It serves us well to know that fasting is not a new practice. Fasting has been used for thousands of years and is one of the oldest therapies in medicine. Many of the great doctors of ancient times and many of the oldest healing systems have recommended it as an integral method of healing and prevention. For example, Ayurvedic medicine, the world's oldest healing system, has long advocated fasting as a major treatment.

In the U.S., the practice of fasting might appear to be a foreign concept, but its use as a curative measure has just as long a history as other medical modalities, including the pills and potions that are so readily touted as primary medical interventions. Fasting has gained popularity in American alternative medicine over the past several decades.

There are many health benefits to fasting. In *How To Eat To Live*, these benefits are clearly stated. First, fasting is the safest and most effective method to detoxify the body. Detoxification is the healing method founded on the principle that toxic substances in the body are responsible for many illnesses and conditions. The Honorable Elijah Muhammad has stated that fasting rids the body of impurities. The blood is cleansed, and as such, is able to better serve the body.

As a detoxification method, fasting has been used to treat nearly every chronic condition, including allergies, anxiety, asthma, depression, diabetes, headaches, heart disease, high cholesterol, low blood sugar, digestive disorders, mental illness, arthritis[2] and obesity.[3] These conditions result from poisons in the body, and from the wear and tear of the organs that result from having to constantly digest food. When our organs are worn through overuse, the digestive process is hindered. This causes disease.

Fasting is also used as a curing method to treat health conditions caused by environmental factors, such as chemical exposure. In several cases, fasting was successfully used to help treat people exposed to high levels of toxic materials, such as polychlorinated biphenyl (PCB) poisoning. [4]

Fasting is one of the best prevention and intervention measures. As an intervention, fasting enables a person to save money rather than expend it. Mainstream medicine, which propagates the use of toxic pills, has caused many to lose their wealth. Those who run this profit-driven industry have successfully painted natural remedies as extreme and unreasonable, and the use of toxic pills and brutal surgical procedures as most realistic.

Reasonably, if anything is stupid or unreasonable (in the truest sense of the word), it is the notion that adding more poison to an already poisoned body can heal a person. This is what pills are—poison. Pills are concentrated chemicals used to combat the sickness caused by an overabundance of chemicals in the body, which in many cases got there through gluttonous eating habits.

In some cases, taking pills to cure disease or sickness is like attempting to put out a gasoline fire by spraying more gasoline on the fire. Pills can play an important role in medical intervention, but they are not capable of healing the body. This is why the Honorable Elijah Muhammad has stated that there is no cure in drugs. If the cause of sickness is due to the poison in the body, then ridding the body of poison and halting the intake of more poison are the best methods of curing the person.

Some people have stated: *If I fast, I will starve to death!* This is not so with fasting as prescribed by the Honorable Elijah Muhammad. He considers going 24 hours without food a fast. Starvation occurs when the body no longer has any stored energy and begins using essential tissues, such as organs, for an energy source. This will not happen in 24 hours. In fact, this will not happen for most people in 3, 4, or 5 days of fasting. Most

2. Sundqvist T, Lindstrom F, Magnusson K, Skoldstam L, Stjernstrom I, Tagesson C. Influence of Fasting on Intestinal Permeability and Disease Activity in Patients with Rheumatoid Arthritis. Scandanavian Journal of Rheumatology 1982;11:33-38.

people in America, a place where the populace is overweight, can afford to take fasts. Some people have plenty of toxic-filled fat to burn away.

The Honorable Elijah Muhammad has pointed out that fasting is a common practice by those who profess membership in the major religions of the world—Christianity, Islam, and Judaism. In religious practices, fasting purifies the mind and heart through abstinence from natural inclinations and urges that keep us tied to the earthly realm of our existence.

In this, fasting allows us to transcend temporal issues and spend more time in the spiritual realm. This is where the soul is fed. We are renewed spiritually and morally, and given the opportunity to put our lives in proper order by reclaiming the true perspective of life's purpose, which is service to God through serving others. There is, however, more to this, as fasting for spiritual growth improves our physical health.

The Honorable Minister Louis Farrakhan has explained that even the root of our physical sickness is spiritual. The spiritual affects and determines (to a recognizable extent) the physical. Current research into the detriments of stress caused by worry and anxiety supports this truth.

Most of us can agree that thinking impacts physical and mental health. We can think ourselves into physical sickness and insanity. Many people have done this and many more continue to place themselves in disease states because of an inordinate view of life, and adverse situations that spring from that view. They are anchored to temporal conditions.

If we look at the concept of fasting as a practice that affords us "total" rest—of the body's organs from the digestive process, and of the mind from the activities and social conditions brought about by an unrighteous world—then we should fast as often as possible for the sake of survival. This is one of the Honorable Elijah Muhammad's recommendations.

3. Kjeldsen-Kragh JH, M; Haugen, M; Forre, O. Antibodies against dietary antigens in rheumatoid arthritis patients treated with fasting and a one-year-vegatarian diet. Clinical and Experimental Rheumatology 1995;13(2):167.

4. Motoo Imamura M, and Ta-Chang Tung, MD. A Trial of Fasting Cure for PCB-Poisoned Patients in Taiwan. American Journal of Industrial Medicine 1984;5:147-153.

8

Doctors Live No Longer Than Patients

Why did the Honorable Elijah Muhammad make the statement: "Doctors do not live longer than their patients".

Superficially, this statement might be taken as mockery; however, the Honorable Elijah Muhammad is not a man who mocks others. Why should He mock anyone? The awesome truths that He has been given, combined with a profound demonstration of these truths in the lives of those who follow him, and through the improved scientific knowledge of this world, shows that His interest is to benefit humanity in the greatest way.

On this note, many people fail to realize that the Honorable Elijah Muhammad's work is at the core of this world's advancement in science. This world's scientific community, however, has neglected and rejected the moral and spiritual truths that are intrinsic to the success of scientific advancements, and by doing this, they have not reaped the great rewards that such scientific advancements would normally bring.

Now, I will answer this question by describing a personal experience that occurred several years ago. While riding the Northeastern Amtrak line from Delaware to New York, I would work on my book, *Nuts Are Not Good For Humans*. The two-hour ride to and from New York gave me the opportunity to get much accomplished. One day, a woman sitting next to me, questioned my writing. I shared my thoughts about nuts—that they are not good for humans to eat.

She disagreed, and responded by pointing out the health-promoting properties of specific elements contained in nuts. I cautioned her about the negative impacts of this type of approach—that the whole food, and not just isolated elements, must be factored in because nutrient-to-nutrient reactions and nutrient-to-digestive enzyme reactions determine the safety of the food.

We wrangled for several minutes. I took her deeper into the biochemistry of nuts and how nuts affect the delicate human digestive tract. I knew my position was thoroughly supported, but she continued to disagree.

Her questioning of me turned personal, as she inquired about my educational training in this field, which I answered correctly by stating that God's Messiah taught me, and that researching His truths has led me to study many life sciences, in my effort to understand and validate those truths.

She finally revealed that she was a certified nutritionist, having a degree from an established university. I thought this interaction very ironic and interesting—that after a lengthy discussion she would reveal her profession.

She further stated that she held a very high position at an institution, where she taught nutrition. She conveyed her experience in helping others through her work. This, as I assessed it, was her trump card to usurp my argument against nuts.

After stating these things, she paused to see my reaction—as if I would retract my position about nuts, or buffer it a little. Of course, I did neither. Besides, it was not my truth to retract. This is Almighty God's truth through His Servant, the Honorable Elijah Muhammad. Through it all, she said nothing that effectively countered the argument against eating nuts.

Now, how would an on-looker decide which one of us is correct? She had the degrees and some work experience. I had God's truth, knowledge of how this truth has saved many lives, and an argument that she failed to refute. What is the most effective deciding factor upon which an on-looker can make the right choice? Where does the ultimate proof rest?

Proof rests in the biological workings that support life. By studying the digestive process, and evaluating the effect of certain foods on this process, we can determine the foods that harm the body. This approach makes the argument against the mainstream recommendations—issued by doctors, nutritionist, and others—effective and victorious.

Fortunately, when it comes to diet and nutrition, the ultimate proof rests in the pudding—the person or people who subscribe to specific diets or boast that they have the correct diet. Does the person's physical appearance and state of health show that he or she has the correct diet? Does the person boasting the right way to eat look like a million dollars or fifty-cents? People can engage the most fantastic and eloquent blathering about diet and nutrition, but at the end of the day, they are judged according to their health status and physical appearance. This is natural.

I cannot fully convey the woman's physical appearance (face, youthfulness, and vitality), but in my honest assessment, she did not look as though she knew anything about nutrition. She was overweight, gray-headed, and noticeably wrinkled. On the other hand, the Honorable Elijah Muhammad's guidance has enabled me to maintain a youthful appearance, and although I was 36 years old at that time, people would often mistake my age for 25 years or younger. If I were the on-looker in this scenario, I would have sided with me. This, however, is not always the case.

Amazingly, some people usually do not see things quite this way. For example, we have often wondered how a 65-year-old person feels when they see the youthfulness and beauty of the Honorable Minister Louis Farrakhan, who is nearly 70 years of age. Does it even occur to that person, that the Minister may know something that he or she does not know? Is there even an eagerness on the part of that person to get involved in the diet that made the Minister look so youthful? It would appear that many people simply pass over this issue, and continue to watch themselves fall to pieces.

Now, if we take my scenario (discussion with the nutritionist on the train) and place it over the medical and health industries, namely those who issue public and personal health advice, then we can better assess who really knows what. The Honorable Elijah Muhammad has done this by pointing out the fact that doctors do not live longer than their patients, as they, too, die at 60, 65, or 70 years of age. They also suffer many years with the very ailments for which they treat others.

This does not mean that their medical training is not valuable. It means that they are in need of proper dietary guidance, as well. This also means that doctors are in no position to tell people that they should not eat one meal a day, as mandated by the Honorable Elijah Muhammad. Many of them know very little about nutrition. Most follow long-held dietary assumptions that have never been substantiated by science. Such is the case with the *three-meals-a-day* nonsense. No scientific proof exist that can justify a human adult eating three or four meals in a single day. Profit, and not the well being of the human family, is the force that drives these lies.

Doctors are just now being encouraged, and in some cases required, to take nutrition courses. For the most part, you can receive a medical degree without having a detailed knowledge of nutrition and diet. This says much about the worth of the dietary advice they give.

Finally, let us revisit this Amtrak experience to drive several other points home. In the context of this example, there are certain aspects we must consider. For example, one can easily tout a certain diet but not adhere to it—making that person an unlikely example of that which they propagate. This could have been the case with that nutritionist, but it was not. How do I know this? Her position was mainstream, which does not have longevity at the base of its nutrition or dietary instruction. If you can locate a nutrition textbook used in universities and colleges that address longevity, including lifespan potentials of 120, 240 or 1,000 years, send it to me. I doubt that one exists.

The subject of longevity is not a hallmark in the mainstream health arena. In fact, it is just the opposite, which is to send us to our graves as quickly as possible. So, her physical degeneration was commensurable with her dietary practices. Under such instructions and practices, youthfulness is impossible to sustain. Nevertheless, she spoke what she believed and lived. She might have been unaware that her physical degeneration, and not her degrees, was the best proof that something was lacking in what she had.

On the other hand, the potential to sustain youthfulness and longevity through the dietary guidance given by the Honorable Elijah Muhammad is immense. This is so whether anyone adheres to it or not. For example, some people do not adhere to this dietary guidance, although they are aware of it and should follow it. The reasons why they do not follow this guidance vary. Unfortunately, such persons are not in the best position to effectively promote *How To Eat To Live*. Why is this so? Again, the proof is always in the pudding. We are required to live that which we apostatize to make our actions or behavior congruent with our words.

A person might state, *"the truth stands on its own so I can still preach it without having to live it"*. To some extent, this is true; however, more must be considered. Truth is to benefit humans and is not something in a vacuum. The truth-giver is just as important and necessary as the truth given, because the truth-giver represents the embodiment and example of that truth.

In this, there is power to motivate an on-looker or prospect to examine or, at least, consider the truth. On the other hand, what motivation would an on-looker have to read *How To Eat To Live* if the physical appearance of the person promoting it is repulsive? Fortunately, the members of the Nation of Islam and their spiritual leader, the Honorable Minister Louis Farrakhan are excellent examples of youthfulness and vitality. They are proof of the power contained in How To Eat To Live to regenerate the human body.

Again, and to conclude, the statement about *doctors not living longer than their patients* does not imply that medical doctors have no value. They have great value. We all know that without medicine and medical practitioners, the trauma caused by careless acts would be unbearable. The Honorable Elijah Muhammad makes this clear.

However, His position is that the enormity of society's health burden should not exist, because much of it is the result of poor dietary habits. By eating correctly, medical situations can be reduced to the fixing of broken bones, sprains and the like, due to falls and accidents.

9

Commercialization

Why does the Honorable Elijah Muhammad state that the intent of this world is to rob, maim, and kill the people for commercialization purposes?

Many people recognize that wickedness, disease, suffering, and death are shockingly pervasive throughout this world. This world epitomizes and confirms the Scriptures where it states that the *"love of money is the root of all evil"*. Evil is the order of the day. Some are aware of the conditions or circumstances that make this world wickedly unbearable. Of course, many people enjoy such a world of folly, sport, play and indecency. For others, this world must go.

The wise people know that in the Scriptures of the Holy Quran and Bible this world is Satan's world. The wise people also know that in the Last Day's pestilence and death intensifies to the point where people begin to wonder if they will make it through because the assault on human life is great. It appears that death is everywhere—that nearly everyone you come across wants to suck life out of you for profit's sake.

The wise people also know that in these Days, Almighty God sends His Servants to save the people or those who would be saved. This salvation is conditional. Those who are saved understand the terrain in which they live and accept the guidance given for their salvation. By terrain, we mean the corrupted systems and destructive ploys of this wicked world. Without knowing the terrain, one is easily victimized.

The Honorable Elijah Muhammad, by alerting us to the treacherous intent of this world's food and health industries to destroy the population, is informing us about the terrain in which we live.[1] These industries are profit-driven.

---

1.   Muhammad E. How To Eat To Live. Chicago: Muhammad's Temple of Islam No. 2, 1972.

In this world, food and health are commercial industries, rather than public or government controlled. Commercialization is defined as: *1) to apply methods of business for profit; 2) to do, exploit, or make chiefly for financial gain; to sacrifice the quality for profit.* Commercialization in these industries is best viewed as a collaboration among those who render false dietary advice, those who manufacture foods, and those who manage healthcare.

As commercial industries, they are profit centers; and as profit centers, sinister mechanisms and machinations are continuously engaged to grab more profit. Here, we must state that this nation's government, although not controlling food distribution and healthcare delivery, construct policies that are supposed to regulate these industries, disallowing them to abuse the population. However, these policies work for the financial benefit of the food and health industries.

These death-dealing merchants reward the government officials who author and support such policies. Obviously, this is not righteous practice, but such is the modi operandi of the governments of this world. Under a righteous government, essential human services are not given over to commerce. Therefore, every person has the essentials of life—food, shelter, and clothing, to name a few. In the U.S., persons with no money do not eat, and people with no health insurance are denied healthcare.

What are the factors that drive us to purchase food? Other than the need for food, false dietary advice, particularly the advocating of eating three meals a day, has most people buying more food than they truly need. Of course, this is important to these profit centers, as they reap untold wealth.

Among these benefits is their influence over our food selection. The public is influenced to eat every despicable creature—insects, creeping-crawling life forms, and poisonous animals. We are also fooled into eating wood-like vegetation and chemical-concocted materials labeled as food. Our adherence to the food industry's every whim, has placed it in a position to make money by putting just about anything on the market. This has also placed us in a volatile position, because nearly everything branded as food threatens our lives.

The danger of commercialization is exacerbated by competition among those who want complete control over the industry. Achieving this control means more power and earning potential for the victor. To date, only a handful of companies control most of the farmland, manufacturing plants, food processing centers and distribution warehouses. Mr. William Robbins sums up the threat caused by this in the book, *The American Food Scandal*:[2]

> The food industry, or agribusiness—the terms are almost interchangeable—has succeeded partly because it has been one of the world's most skillful practitioners of the technique of the big lie. Americans, we are told, are blessed with better food at lower costs than anyone in any other country. So we are told by the industry, which is the world's largest concentration of financial power. We are told so by the industry's lobbyists, who compose the most potent political force in Washington. And their message is chorused by Congressmen and bureaucrats in the national capital who guard the industry's interests and do its bidding.

These deceitful dealings should come as no surprise to most people. Money, as the chief source of security in this world, and the prize of nearly everyone, means that we should expect little or no integrity from those who claim to represent the people. The deplorable condition of the populace is proof of the satanic behavior of politicians and evidence of their failed commitment to serve the people. The atmosphere of inordinate self-interest is very apparent. Mr. Robbins continues:

> Our food is grown, processed and impregnated with chemicals, with hardly a passing thought from the industry about their effect on the consumer's health and little show of concern when an ingredient, after long use, turns out to be carcinogenic.

Of course, the situation has changed dramatically since 1974, when this book was published. Since that time the inordinate greed of the *merchants of death*, combined with the gradual and continuous chastisement of Almighty God on this land, has sent the *merchants of death* to chemical laboratories to concoct foods. In some cases, we consume more manufactured chemicals than we do God-made foods. The Honorable Minister Louis Farrakhan wrote in his great book, *A Torchlight for America*:[3]

---

2. Robbins W. The American Food Scandal 'Why You Can't Eat Well on What You Earn. New York: Willliam Morrow & Company, Inc., 1974.
3. Farrakhan ML. A Torchlight for America. Chicago: FCN Publishing Co., 1993

The food industry is a $400 billion industry, based on promoting death-dealing, overly processed foods...The foods get difibered, degerminated, defatted, refatted, and manipulated in countless ways other than how food is intended for us to eat. It's no coincidence that the first heart attack reported in America was in 1896, the same time our diets began changing from a rural-based local supply of foods to national food supply chains of highly processed foods.

We must note that in 1997, Americans spent $715 billion for food and another $95 billion for alcoholic beverages.[4] History records that the turn of the nineteenth century brought about tremendous changes in food processing as urbanization began to mold the "new" America. Other ways to preserve foods came into demand as the transition from rural-based and local food supply shifted to national food manufacturing and distribution. Obviously, this shift also brought about changes in food quality, as well as changes to the overall health of consumers. One historical perspective states:[5]

Food was commonly adulterated for economic gain in both Europe and the United States in the 1800s...Harvey Wiley, a U.S. Department of Agriculture (USDA) chemist, campaigned against the common practices of adulterating foods and published a number of articles and pamphlets on the subject. He was in part responsible for the passage of food laws and the establishment of the U.S. Food and Drug Administration which to this day has the responsibility for preventing adulteration of foods in the United States.

Of course, much can be stated about the FDA's failure to uphold its responsibility. By every feasible account, the FDA is a greater proponent of commercialization and exploitation than it is a protector and defender of the American public.

The pervasive false and dangerous dietary advice, combined with chemical-concocted foods, is responsible for the chronic disease epidemic. This epidemic is the lifeblood of the healthcare industry, and has been such for centuries. This profit center harnesses trillions of dollars through this epidemic.[6] How could the healthcare industry generate profits

4.   Putnam JJ, Allshouse JE. Food Consumption, Prices, and Expenditures, 1970-97. Washington, D.C.: Economic Research Service (ERS), USDA, 1999.
5.   Olsen JBaWC, ed. The Contemporary And Historical Literature Of Food Science And Nutrition. Ithaca: Cornell University Press, 1995.

unless there was an unhealthy population to treat? The *merchants of death* are committed to keeping us sick and diseased so they can hurl poisonous pills, potions, and bogus research at us night and day. There is no letup because the drive for profit has reached extreme madness.

The Honorable Elijah Muhammad, by giving us the truth of this world's treachery in the food and healthcare industries, has identified our enemies. Knowing the aim of this world, and all its colorful pitfalls, enables us to be in the world but not of it. This is salvation, and is a point that we must examine.

The most readily acceptable meaning of *not being of the world* is the participation in church, mosque, or synagogue services throughout the week. But during the rest of the week, the same people partake of every activity presented to them by this world—Satan's world. They eat forbidden foods, such as swine flesh; drink wine and whiskey; smoke cigarettes and dope; and lie and steal.

The same people also accept the guidance of this world's leaders, and support demonic war efforts to bomb, murder, and maim other peoples. This way of life is certainly *being of the world*, as taking mere oaths and attending religious worship services account for little or nothing.

Meanwhile, the truth is rejected because of gross ignorance among the people. This behavior prevents many people from truly living the quality of life that Almighty God intends, which is the new way of life given to us through the Honorable Elijah Muhammad and the Honorable Minister Louis Farrakhan. This new way of life caters to every human need— freedom, justice, equality, proper human relationships, fair economics, health, diet, spirituality, etc. No stone is unturned. The *life* given to us through the Honorable Elijah Muhammad is one that goes far beyond the mere singing of songs and verbal worship of the Almighty God.

This *life* is *not of this world*, although it is *lived* in this world. It is a *saved life* because Satan is unable to destroy it for profit's sake.

---

6.   Statistics NCfH. Health, United States, 2001, with Urban and Rural Health Chartbook. Hyattsville, Maryland: Department of Health and Human Services, Centers for Disease Control and Prevention, 2001.

Index